TH PERFE MYTH

How to Break Free From the Dogmatic Chains of Health and Dieting

By: Madelyn Moon

www.maddymoon.com

Publishing services provided by Archangel Ink

ISBN: 1942761651
ISBN-13: 978-1-942761-65-5

Table of Contents

A Letter to the Reader

Hi, beautiful.

I'm really glad you decided to pick up this book today.

In case you were curious, I'll go ahead and tell you up front. *The Perfection Myth* is going to call you to be vulnerable and honest with yourself. If you believe that achieving "ideal" aesthetics is the key to happiness, than this book found you for a reason. This topic is scary, sure. It's not something many of us *want* to come to terms with.

The truth is, our relationship with our body can hinder us from chasing after our life's purpose. We are so attached to our physical ideals because they are comfortable. They are something we can work towards. But they are also distracting, unrealistic, hindering and even damaging. They are damaging to both the mind and the body because they lead you to see yourself as less than who you are. You can become so entirely consumed with your body in hopes that it will change, that you miss out on the beautiful creation it is, and the beautiful things it can do.

My whole intention with this book is to teach you how you can heal your mind-body relationship and learn how to block out the perfectionist nonsense distributed by your peers, family, and the media today.

In this book, I'm going to share my personal story about how I used to damage my body out of fear and how I eventually reinvented myself out of love. I am going to be vulnerable, and I hope you can be, too.

I am going to tell you about the myth that lies all around us. *The Perfection Myth.*

With that said, I'm not saying I have everything figured out in regard to my food choices or my mind-body relationship. I'm not saying, "Oh, praise Jesus, I'm completely and utterly in love with everything about me, and acceptance is so easy, and I'm so happy to be free from all food and body dilemmas!"

Uh, no, and I can almost promise you that if anybody says that, they're most likely fibbing to some degree, no matter how small. Having a bad day here and there is completely normal.

Some important things I hope you learn in this book are:

- Perfection isn't real.
- You shouldn't look up to the media as inspiration.
- Disordered eating goes way deeper than what meets the eye.
- Confidence is golden.
- Nutrition is about what works best for you and *only* you.
- Fitness doesn't have to be complicated.
- Your full potential is waiting to burst out. All you have to do is give it permission to do so.

Throughout this book, we're going to discuss the above topics and many more.

I'm also going to provide you with some self-loving practices that will improve your current quality of life.

Nothing is going to happen overnight, so stick with me.

I'm actually trying to teach you some pretty intense things. Things most women don't learn until much later in life. You're going to learn how to recognize and experience your true potential *now*, rather than later. You're going to learn how to finally *love* your body. You're going to learn how to seek satisfaction and self-worth in places other than your physical appearance.

These are not easy lessons to learn, my friends. But if you're up for the challenge, I am too.

With love,

Madelyn

1

My Story

L et's get something straight.
My story is not a woe-is-me, poor helpless me, little ole me needs sympathy kind of story.

This is a *"you're not alone story."*

If you struggle with body image or disordered eating, you may feel like you're the only person in the world who is suffering so intensely, but the truth is, it's all around. And I think it's time we do something to feel less alone and to heal our bodies and hearts.

That's where my book comes into play. And hence, here we are in Chapter One, talking about me—the most uncomfortable subject I'll write about in this entire book, but arguably one of the most important.

If you're not interested in learning about my pre-discovery life, feel free to skip this chapter and go straight to Chapter 2. Otherwise, get ready because I'm about to get real.

HIGH SCHOOL

I have memories of being concerned with my body before high school, if I'm being completely honest. The first memory I own of recognizing the relationship between food and weight is when I was watching an innocent children's television show where the main character's best friend was living under stressful conditions and decided that starving herself from food was the best way to deal with life's hard times.

Light bulb.

Though I was in my early teens, I had never realized before that controlling my food and weight would be the "perfect" distraction from uncomfortable obstacles thrown my way. Even though the show ended with her best friend realizing starvation was silly and wrong, that's not the message I received. I had learned something new and exciting, and no matter how "sorry" her best friend was, I was curious and interested.

Fast-forward a few years and we've landed in high school. As a tenth grader, I had a best friend who was vegan. Several documentaries and tofu scrambles later, I conformed to all-or-nothing vegetarianism with strong ethical beliefs. Pair this with my compulsive nature and you've got a very unbalanced chick.

During this time, I was also hanging with a lot of athletes. I was very conscious about the fact that my body did not look like theirs. I was pretty lean, but I was what they call (ugh, I hate this stupid phrase) "skinny fat."

Please keep in mind this is one of the most curious times of my entire life. I asked complete strangers how they got "so skinny" and listened to them rave about their afternoon elliptical ventures.

I asked girlfriends how they got such flat stomachs and immediately tried out their 30-minute abdominal circuit rituals.

I watched free workouts on television and spent my days reading fitness magazines for the best fat-blasting workouts. I distinctly remember doing this really odd sit-up holding a broom and letting one foot go over and under the broom, followed by the other foot, for at least 100 reps a day.

As I was trying out all of these strange new exercise techniques, I was also exploring my new diet. Though I originally started vegetarianism for ethical reasons, my mission became overpowered by my desire to look lean and perfect.

Most of the food I ate consisted of 80-calorie yogurts, white bread, low fat crackers, and peanut butter.

Gah, I ate so much peanut butter.

Eating this way, I definitely did not get "fat," but I also wasn't reaching my physique goals. This was so frustrating to me.

Cue the no eating at all phase

This one was rough but short-lived. And it's a good time to mention that in this book, I will never say that I had an eating disorder…because I didn't. What I will say is that I had disordered eating.

For example, there were a few days I would see how long I could go without eating, as I kept up with my workouts. I distinctly remember one time I went four days without so much as a bite of food. I have no idea how I could have possibly done this considering high school is already stressful enough, but I did it. And this story ends with me passing out at a friend's house, hitting my head on her door on the way down, and having her mom call my parents to come pick me up. After I was fed with a decent helping of yogurt and bread, that is.

That was the last time I tried that. It was humiliating and obviously not working.

COLLEGE

My time in college was great for the most part. Similar to most people, I really didn't realize how good I had it until I graduated.

I spent two years at the University of Arkansas in Fayetteville and two years at the University of Texas at Austin. Both were very different experiences, and I appreciate them both tremendously.

Let's start with my time at University of Arkansas.

I joined a sorority from the beginning and had the time of my life. Parties, boys, drinking, new friends, new classes, etc. All was really good, except for the fact that I was treating my body like crap.

I drank too much, I ate too little, and I "worked out" way more than I should have. My workouts consisted of spending an hour on the elliptical or the treadmill until I burnt 1,000 calories and then doing my trusty 30-minute abdominal circuit. Afterwards, I would go back to my dorm to refuel on white bread and peanut butter.

I was doing it so, so, so wrong on so many levels.

The thing I did MOST wrong here was hate my body. I was not running on the treadmill for hours a day out of respect and love for myself...I was running because of the fear I possessed about what would happened if I stopped running. It came from a place of obsession.

If you're running an hour a day on the treadmill out of love and enjoyment, that's one thing. Seriously, more power to you. Don't think I'm putting those activities down at all. I'm merely describing my attitude during those activities, and they were not pretty at all.

At the University of Arkansas, I got into a nasty habit of drinking too much on the weekends, getting sick, sleeping for a couple hours, and then going to the gym to run bright and early (even if I was still a little tipsy). It was a compulsive routine.

Every morning I had the same schedule. I would wake up, go for my run, and then afterwards, I would check out my stomach. I would rate how flat it was on a scale from 1-10 based on the previous day. Did I look smaller? Bigger?

The crazy thing is, I had actually lost 15 pounds my freshman year from my unhealthy relationship with my body. I had a lot of work to do.

Fast-forward a bit.

I "found myself" in my sophomore year and started to lay off the obsessions just a little. I lived in the sorority house and spent more time with my friends, searching for answers about how to love myself more. I was still partying a bit more than I should have, but I was trying to find some sort of balance.

Soon enough, I decided that I wanted to move to Austin, Texas. I had visited it once my freshman year and had fallen in love. I submitted my application to the University of Texas and received an envelope a few months later with my acceptance letter inside. Without a second thought, I packed up and moved back to my home state.

My time at the University of Texas was interesting on so many levels. I was no longer in a sorority, so I had to really work to make new friends.

I partied a little bit, but I became more interested in the bodybuilding lifestyle than anything.

I began to see these pictures of the women I wanted to look like—those women with tan bodies, stage-ready abs, perfect booties, and gloriously symmetrical muscles.

And just like that, I knew what my next goal was.

I read up on bodybuilding diets and realized I was doing it all wrong. I put down my tempeh and carrots and picked up a plate of chicken and broccoli. It seemed like the right thing to do at the time.

I had quickly fallen into the trap so many of us do. I looked at these women and their perfectly sculpted bodies and thought they had to be happier than me. I assumed they had more in life. They exemplified perfection in every area of their lives. I wanted that.

I hired my first bodybuilding coach, and he put me on a 1400-calorie diet with workouts that lasted at least two hours. The diet I was prescribed stuck around for the entire four-month prep. And when I say that diet stuck around, I literally mean that exact diet. Nothing changed.

Not a blueberry more or a spinach leaf less.

I thought that if I ate an ounce more than my meal plan told me to, I wouldn't win the show. That's how intense my focus was.

In my mind, "balance" meant allowing myself to have an Emergen-C packet once a week. You know which ones I'm talking about? The immunity building packets you pour in water when you're fighting a cold?

Yeah, I would eat those straight from the packet. They were my dessert. And I still felt guilty afterwards, as if those five calories were going to ruin my chances of finally obtaining that perfect body.

Gross.

Hopefully by now you're getting the picture. I was extremely consumed by my appearance; so much so that I couldn't even enjoy the little things in life, like being young.

Now let's talk about the physical torture my body was going through and some of the things that happen when your body is in a severe state of stress.

Number one, I lost my period.

This is one of the first things to go when your body is under a tremendous amount of stress. Your body must conserve energy where it can, and since reproduction isn't an absolute necessity, it's the first thing to go.

Number two, I was really gassy. I think this came from a combination of things. I didn't poop much because I was lacking fiber, dietary fat, and things that help poop "move" along. I was also eating a high-protein diet, which can cause gas in some people. On top of these things, I was digesting food in an anxious state, and yes, that too can cause gas.

Truth be told, a lot of the lean people you see in magazines are suffering from a tremendous amount of gas and bloat because their bodies aren't sure how to digest and process it all.

I couldn't even tell you how many times I left a room with people to go "relieve" myself in the bathroom. It happened way too often than I'd like to confess.

Number three, I couldn't poop. I already said this one, but I really want to emphasize it. Not being able to poop for several days in a row causes a lot of buildup and bloat, and this is not easy for a self-conscious person to deal with, especially when you're dying to be lean all the time. I cried and cried and cried many nights because I was so backed up and looked so bloated.

Has this ever happened to you? Poop problems suck.

Number four, I lost sleep. Being able to sleep throughout the night is a solid measure for health. If you're waking up multiple times during your rest, you may need to think about your stress levels, including both your mental and physical health. Both of those were going down the drain for me, and so my sleep was suffering big time. As a result, I started taking Tylenol PM and Advil PM to get to sleep. Soon enough, I was addicted.

SHOW TIME

The actual bodybuilding show I had spent four months dieting for had finally arrived.

I felt ready.

Granted, I was the smallest one competing, but I was fairly confident in my transformation.

I had my spray tan, my bedazzled green suit, and my family there to support me. I went on the stage with full confidence, strutted my stuff, and found myself placing 9th out of 20.

What?!

I didn't see that coming. I thought all my dieting would have paid off. I thought that this would be my moment of sheer satisfaction. This was the night I had spent four months working towards.

But one of the most interesting things was that even the second and third place winners did not look happy. They were upset because they didn't get first. They were upset because it wasn't enough.

They didn't feel like *they* were enough.

It was never enough.

I'm going to say something that may get me in trouble with some true bodybuilding believers…but I really think even the first place winners didn't feel satisfied. They wouldn't be satisfied until the next show. But wait, no, satisfaction will come from the next show after that. No? Okay, maybe the next!

And the cycle continues.

The reason why people are never truly satisfied after a period of weight loss is because *self-worth cannot be found in aesthetics.*

Happiness will never be uncovered by changing the size and shape of your glutes or the smallness of your waist. Happiness is only found within, and when you let yourself believe otherwise, the desire to change your already amazing body will become overpowering.

I was starting to discover this.

I didn't completely accept that lesson until the next year, to be honest. I had signed up to do another show, and the night of *that* show was when I really, truly accepted the fact that I needed to change.

(I know what you're thinking. "Madelyn, you're crazy! Wasn't one enough!?")

I went through the starvation, the overtraining, the anxiety, the lack of sleep, the relationship-deprived nights, and then the self-loathing thoughts all over again.

I kept thinking, *I can do this. If I quit, I'm a failure. People think I'm some sort of fitness super star; I can't let them down. I have to prove that I can win!*

The second show was awful. I had a horrible time. I was disappointed in my placing, and I was such a party pooper (minus the pooping).

To be honest, I believe this was a great thing. I think that if I had actually placed better in the rankings and had a good time, I would have still been hooked in this terrible cycle. I consider myself lucky to have had such a terrible, eye-opening experience.

The night after the show, I was lying in my hotel bedroom with my family, and I said aloud, "Mom, this wasn't worth it. None of this was worth the costs and sacrifices."

I'm sure it probably sounded like I was talking about the food sacrifices, but I was actually talking about my mental health. I was tired of hating myself. I was tired of only seeing the bad in my body. I was frustrated that there were people out there that were 20 pounds heavier than me but so much happier.

I was so tired of fearing food and fearing the scale. I knew something needed to change.

That night is what I would call my "aha" moment. That's the evening I truly felt like my attitude and feelings towards myself had hit rock bottom.

POST COLLEGE

I finished up college and moved.

As much as I love Austin, TX, I wasn't being the person I knew I needed to be there. I was too self-consumed, and there was a small little voice in my head saying things would be different if I just went to Colorado.

A Texas girl in the Mile High City.

A week after this thought popped in my head, I made the commitment. I packed up my bags and my newly adopted puppy and hit the road.

I didn't tell many people. I felt that slipping away unannounced might be my best tactic.

Moving to Colorado was the best thing I ever could have done for myself. It didn't happen overnight, but escaping the body-conscious culture I found myself trapped in in Austin did amazing things for my self-worth.

I started living differently. I became kinder to myself. I started to trust my intuition again (with a lot of hard work). I created friendships that were genuine and insightful. I looked at mountains and beauty daily.

I stopped believing in perfection and started experiencing gratitude for who I was, regardless of the external world's views.

I'm not going to pretend that my journey to self-discovery was easy by any means. There were some crying fits, some calorie counting, some meal planning, and some food anxiety.

With that said, I have finally experienced food freedom and body respect. You may have heard that it's possible before but never actually believed it. Well, I'm here to say they were right…it *is* possible.

It might not be easy. But it is possible.

The rest of this book is going to focus on how you too can discover yourself, create unconditional body respect, and finally find food freedom.

2

Perfection is Subjective

Part of *The Perfection Myth* is to challenge social norms and explore freedom in more ways than one. Letting go of perfection means to let go of the "perfect" weight, but also the *idea* that there is a perfect weight.

For example, I used to believe it was possible to find happiness by changing my body.

Until I tried to achieve it.

For your own general knowledge, the definition of perfection is as follows:

The condition, state, or quality of being free or as free as possible from all flaws or defects.

Oh, okay, so perfection involves a state of physical freedom. Well, what does freedom mean?

The state of not being imprisoned or enslaved.

Well, isn't that interesting. By definition, to be perfect means to be free of defects, and to be free means to not be enslaved. Wouldn't it make sense then that being perfect means to not be enslaved?

What happens when your desire to achieve that perfection means that you're anything but free? That, in reality, you're completely enslaved?

Also, where are those defects listed out?

How can we possibly know what exactly is a defect, where it is created, and where it lives?

What does a defect look like? What does having one mean for us? Enslavement?

The concept of perfection is confusing. In order to minimize this confusion, the media took the reins and decided for us what perfection was going to look like. They built a multibillion-dollar industry by defining perfection. Nobody else could, so why not them, the nation's biggest influencers?

This is how it's been for centuries; it's the same way we know what is "in" for spring and "out" for fall. We listen to the media and wait for Hollywood to tell us how to look, how to dress, what to eat, and, simply put, how to live.

It's very likely that up until this point you've subconsciously been taking advice from complete and total strangers on who you should be. You may be aware that they are the reason you are so dissatisfied with your body, but you may not be aware of the extent of that dissatisfaction.

I'm going to share a story with you.

There was once a time in my life where I was driven to pain and anguish due to self-criticism. Every morning I would lift up my shirt to analyze my abs, or lack thereof, and that's how I started my day.

And then there was a midday check. And a nightly check (of course, that was never satisfying, considering by then I had pounds of bloat-inducing veggies in me).

But yet, I couldn't stop looking. It was as if I had to check to see if they were there yet; if they had suddenly made an appearance. And when they didn't, I would beat myself up about it and dwell on this so-called flaw of mine (in the weight-loss advertisement industry, everybody has abs, so you begin to think it's mandatory...or at least "the norm").

Let me tell you about the time I realized my lack of abs (or in my mind, a "flaw") was normal, beautiful, and unique.

When you participate in a fitness show, you have to get a ridiculous tan. And if you sign up to be tanned by whatever tanning company is sponsoring the show, it's very likely you will be *nakie* with a lot of other competitors.

So for my last competition, I went in for my scheduled appointment and was in a room with four other girls.

All naked. All lean. And all "fit."

No, I'm not going to tell you I was sad and discouraged because they all looked so amazing, blah blah blah.

I'm actually going to say this: *they all had flaws.*

Yes, they all had flaws. Completely uncovered, naked and bare.

In actuality, it was beautiful.

Here all of us were, competing to get a high ranking on a stage for our physical attributes...but beneath all of the Lululemon, Athleta, and Nike, we all have real, imperfect skin.

And it's all different.

I can't really go into detail about everything I saw, but it was a wide range of everything.

Stretch marks, awkwardly placed moles, skin spots, different shaped breasts, bruises, cuts, burns, odd you-know-whats...you name it, I saw it.

You see, after we put on our custom-made suits with extra bodacious boobie pads, apply our sparkly and dramatic stage makeup, hire a professional photographer, and get our tans, waxes, French nails, and everything else, it's pretty easy to cover up all those "flaws."

It's the same way Photoshop can make you lose ten pounds in a jiff.

Remember, I'm NOT discrediting any of these women, or myself, for the hard work we put into each and every show. I'm merely pointing out something that you may never have thought about.

In fact, I never really thought about that either. Until I saw it for myself. I saw how real each and every one of us is. We are so unique, so imperfect, and so vulnerable.

It definitely took precedence in my mind during my last show.

It made me take a step back and think about the things on my body I consider flawed. I immediately think about my tummy, because it's so hard for me to reach and then maintain that level of leanness.

But...that's so incredibly normal.

We as women are built to have extra body fat for reproduction. Our hormones make sure of it. Our fat distribution has a purpose.

And if it's not a tummy thing for you, it may be something else. You may not completely enjoy your knuckles. Or that freckle on your left boob. Or your nose may not be "ideal."

Again, that's normal. If we were all the same, how boring would that be?

You were created a certain way for a reason.

You are not flawed in any way, shape, or form. In fact, flaws are subjective in the same way that perfection is subjective. Flaws and perfection don't have any clear criteria or boundaries; ultimately, neither is real.

3

The Media is Not Your Role Model

Most of us think perfection is real, simply because we see the same thing on the television every day (e.g., flat stomachs, straight noses, curvy butts) and start to THINK that this type of perfection is not only tangible, but also practical.

But it's not. It's just what gets the most attention.

The reason why the media shows us the same image, the same definition of beauty time and time again is because they need to support and grow their multibillion-dollar industries, such as the diet, plastic surgery, and beauty industries.

When was the last time you saw a commercial promoting *just* inner beauty? (And don't say the Dove commercials because even still, a world class Photoshop professional edited those.)

Think about it: When was the last time you saw a model that looked like an awkward sixteen-year-old? I mean seriously, even the Old Navy kids are free of the inconvenient pimples that most kids have.

Simply said, we are never marketed what we already have or what we naturally look like.

Why? Because this message says you are already complete. It says, "We give up, there's really nothing you need to buy because you're already pretty great."

And where does this lead them?

Nowhere.

No longing factor = no income.

But on the flip side, if they consistently remind us of the seduction factor and glamour that we're *lacking,* well then, they will be making so much money they won't know what to do with it.

This is why a less-than-optimal body image and the desire to be perfect are almost inescapable. It's surrounding us, and we're taught from a young age that THIS is what beauty looks like. THIS is what happy people look like. THIS is what successful people look like.

So now that I've made it pretty clear that this lie is everywhere, it may seem impossible to avoid it.

But that's not true.

There's one practice I've developed that has really, really changed the way I see media…to the point that it no longer affects my day-to-day inner thoughts or reflections on myself.

What I do is this: I challenge EVERYTHING I am told via media about beauty.

Back in the day when I decided to start doing this, I realized that I didn't believe what the mainstream had to say about science-based nutrition (umm, egg yolks are bad, what?), so why was I letting them influence my perception of beauty?

How can the media determine something so intensely subjective when they were so clearly wrong about things that were based on cold hard facts?

It was clear. I needed to start from scratch.

I had to determine for myself what it means to be beautiful if I ever wanted to accept my own unique beauty.

This is my challenge to you: *Define beauty for yourself, and I promise, your outlook on the world around you, as well the world within you, will change forever.*

In order to start this process, one of the best things you can do is clear yourself from the media for a while. It's hard to make progress with anything if you're constantly being reminded and convinced of the opposite thing.

The second best thing you can do is to verbally relay the beliefs you are developing to other people when the opportunity arises.

Many times when people tell me that they "feel fat," I ask them, what does "feeling fat" feel like? And then I listen as they try to scramble together a reason, though it becomes apparent to them that feeling fat feels like insecurity.

In passing, sometimes my girlfriends will comment on the weight loss of another person in admiration but then will quickly add a comment that leads me to believe they are feeling emotions like jealousy. At this point, I usually ask them what this person actually *has* that they do not. Usually, they can come up with nothing.

When I speak up about people that I admire, I no longer say, "Oh my gosh, I love you, you are so pretty." Instead, I speak the truth. I say exactly why I love them.

They always leave me feeling so confident.

They radiate health.

They are beautiful both on the inside and outside.

And so on.

These two practices have helped both me and my clients come to terms with our own bodies because we start to see the beauty of others' making magic IN their body, not just on the OUTSIDE of their body.

4

Sexiness is Already Inside of You

One common reason people want to look lean, lose weight, and improve their bodies is to look sexier.

Looking sexier results in *feeling* sexier.

Right?

The truth is, sexiness has absolutely nothing to do with appearance.

Really, it doesn't.

Sexiness has everything to do with confidence. Sexiness starts on the inside and, as a result, radiates on the outside.

You know a confident person when you see her because she is sexy.

She walks with courage, and she talks with bravery. She uses her talents to help others because she knows her value and her self-worth.

She is confident in her relationships because she has chosen to spend her time with people who lift her up and encourage her to be her own best version of herself.

She does not spend time with people who are lacking ambition or dreams because she does not want to be negatively influenced.

She believes that beauty is not something you're born with; it's something you create.

She knows that no amount of calorie counting or macronutrient timing will bring her happiness.

She knows that the man of her dreams is as fortunate to have her as she is to have him.

She knows that she should feed her body with nutrient-rich foods so that it will perform at its best.

She moves her body; she does not "work out."

She speaks with intention and does not waste time speaking to those who do not listen.

She has an open heart and an open mind.

She is always eager to learn from those who have experience to share.

She knows that looks will fade but confidence never does.

She is confident in everything she does.

In the same way that beauty is not something you are simply born with, neither is confidence. Life has a funny way of bringing us down, and sometimes it's not simple to pick yourself back up.

Fortunately, no matter what trials you experience, they will pass. And you will learn something from each and every one. Together, these small trials are what make you a confident woman.

Through and through, the one and only "trick" behind becoming a confident and sexy woman is this—*self-trust*.

If I could teach you one thing in this entire book, I would want you to know that you should never apologize for being you. If you can learn to trust yourself and never feel ashamed of your inner beauty, then your outer beauty will shine forth so much more powerfully. So many of the small nagging things consuming your mind will disintegrate.

If you can learn to trust yourself, you will:

- *Be so much more confident.* You know there isn't a good reason in this world to be ashamed.
- *Easily forgive yourself when something doesn't go according to plan.* You know you can learn something from EVERY experience.
- *Make decisions with ease.* You have your own instinct for a reason.

- *Never settle.* You know what you need in your life, and you won't stop until it's yours.
- *Allow your body to take its natural shape.* You realize there is no point in trying to force your body to look like somebody else's.

Being a confident, sexy woman starts with self-trust.

It starts with believing that you have something unique to offer this world and that you were created to supply just that.

As much as I hate to say it, no matter who you are, people will always try to dim your light.

There will be people who want to discourage you from creating greatness, from being great.

Sometimes it's the people that are closest to you that discourage you the most. Whether it's out of fear, insecurity, anger, jealousy, or envy, they *will* find a reason to speak up and share their doubt.

Being a confident, sexy woman does not mean that you do not ever doubt yourself, because we all do at times. What it means is that you do not let doubt stop you.

Confident women understand that people will try to bring them down, the world will try to destroy them, and their own self-doubt will frequently get in the way.

But confident women also know that there is no greater fear than fear itself, and there is absolutely no reason to hold back their absolute full potential.

Many times, I made the mistake of believing that sexiness could be created or destroyed by my external appearance.

Like so many women, I thought my beauty (and confidence) was as fragile as glass. It could be gone in a minute if I ate the wrong foods or I missed too many workouts. I spent so much time working on my physical perfection in hopes that confidence would finally come forth that I never experienced even a spark of confidence within me.

Truth.

At my leanest, I was at my least confident.

I had no ambitions, no thriving relationships, and absolutely no love life. I thought that if I finally had the body that "men wanted," then I would finally have the life that I *wanted*.

Once I finally had that perfect body that I thought men wanted, I couldn't even hold a conversation because I was so deprived of dietary fat. I was so consumed with my body that I couldn't go on any dates to show it off. I was pinching pennies because I was trying to afford all my monthly supplements and food.

Most of all, I was so insecure I didn't think I was worthy of going on a date.

I thought I still had work to do on my body. I still needed to change a few things here and there before I allowed myself to indulge in date food.

I was trying to create confidence in all the wrong ways.

Today I have experienced what it means to be truly confident. The moment I realized that my body will never supply me with confidence is the moment I realized that confidence had to be discovered elsewhere. It had to be created through my internal beliefs.

I had to believe that I was confident NOW, not that I would be confident only THEN.

This of course did not happen overnight, but once I started to use all of the practices I go over in this book, I began to not only feel confident, but more important, I believed I had every reason in the world to be confident.

And this, my friends, is why I am sexy.

5

Making All Kinds of Sense Out of Disordered Eating

DISORDERED EATING AND FEAR

There are multiple reasons why we decide to take our emotions out on our food.

The top six reasons are as follows:

- We're not okay with our weight.
- We're uncomfortable with the unknown/lack of control.
- We're afraid.
- We have a Type A personality.
- We trust everyone but ourselves.
- We need a distraction.

Let's take a deeper look at these.

Reason number one, we're not okay with our weight.

Contrary to common sense, it's not always about controlling the food.

So many of us find ourselves obsessing over food, calories, and macronutrients because we are actually obsessing over our weight. We are trying to keep our weight under control.

If you have an incredible weight loss story, maybe you're worried you'll gain weight again.

If you went on a diet for five months before your wedding pictures and had amazing results, maybe you're terrified your husband won't love you as much with a little weight added back on.

Maybe you have absolutely no reason to obsess over your weight but simply can't stop.

You are doing this for a reason. You are focusing on your weight for a reason. You are trying to control your size for a reason.

This ties in with reason number two. *You are trying to control the uncontrollable. You are afraid of what will happen without the ability to control the outcome.*

At this time, I want to ask you as a reader to be open and vulnerable as you think about what I'm about to tell you. Try to apply it to your own life and see if this rings true for you.

- *Has an experience triggered deep-seated fear in you?*
- *Has an event caused you to desire control over all things unknown?*
- *Can you remember a moment that changed the course of the rest of your life?*

I can. I have experienced many moments that have "set me off" and made me cling to my magazine clippings of fitness models, run to my treadmill, and barricade myself indoors on Friday nights so that I could punish myself for that cake I ate *the week before*.

I decided that I wasn't okay with life, so therefore I wasn't okay with my weight, and ultimately that led me to decide I would never be "okay" with the food that went into my body.

It's all a cycle, you see. How you feel about your life is correlated to how you feel about your body. Your fixation on eating, or a lack of eating, is simply a result of that fear of weight gain; it's not necessarily about the food. It's about the weight.

Having something like food to fixate over is:

- A distraction
- A coping mechanism
- A comfort
- A ritual

When life starts to feel out of control, oftentimes it's this distraction that brings us the most comfort.

We think to ourselves, "Well, my job couldn't get any more stressful than it is right now, so I'll just starve myself to make it go away."

Or maybe you think, "Well, he never asked me out on a date, so maybe I am too big. Yes, I will start a diet tomorrow because THEN I know he won't be able to resist me."

As a human being, we think that when something is out of our hands, we should find something else to focus on that is in our hands. Some of us choose alcohol abuse, some choose sex abuse, some choose violence, and then there are many of us who choose self-sabotaging techniques, both physical and mental.

This takes us to reason number three: *Fear*. Being able to control the controllable is one of the most satisfying but self-destructive experiences you will ever have if it comes from a place of fear.

You will never win this battle.

So what should you do instead?

You have two options.

1. Change what's going on around you.
2. Change what's going on within you.

This is the part where I get real with you about your disordered eating. I am about to tell you a truth you may not want to hear. Are you ready?

YOU MIGHT NOT BE LIVING THE LIFE YOU NEED TO BE LIVING.

You may be so extremely uncomfortable with what's happening around you that it's creating a domino effect and morphing what's going on within you. You may hate your body *because* you hate your life.

Change your life and…you won't ever need to change your body.

If your life isn't going the way you planned, you will never EVER create the life you DID plan for by controlling what you eat for dinner or what your scale says in the morning. Ever.

You need to take action. This will mean that you might need to face some extremely uncomfortable situations.

- It might be time to break up with him.
- It might be time to leave your job.
- It might be time to dismiss her from your life.
- It might be time to get rid of *things* you've had lying around that remind you of whomever.
- It might be time to become more spiritual.
- It might be time to forgive yourself for your past.
- It might be time to forgive *them* for their past.
- It might be time to give yourself permission to be you.

I implore you to look at the list above and evaluate your own current situation.

Are you honestly happy with everything in your life? Are you spending time with people who make you a better person?

If not, and if you're trying to control your weight as a result of it, it's time that you put an end to it.

It doesn't happen overnight, but you can certainly start taking action steps today to create the life that you want tomorrow.

And the beautiful thing about changing your external situation is that it can result in an internal realization.

If the root of your stress is grounded in an external factor, then simply subtracting it from your life can result in inner peace and satiety.

Reason number four behind disordered eating: *you may have a Type A personality.*

This type of person is easily influenced by their desire to go all out in everything they do. This type of person might believe that moderation is for sissies or that anything less than 100% is the same as weakness.

This person's eating disorder might possibly just be a result of their Type A qualities. They may need to have something to focus on at all times because they want to *belong somewhere.*

There is something about belonging to a group of people that all prevail or all suffer or all conquer or all XYZ together that makes them believe an all-or-nothing attitude is actually a good thing. It's unfortunate if they choose to focus on food, but it's also very common because many people do create groups based on their diets.

If you're somebody who is suffering from disordered eating because you have a Type A personality, pay attention to all of the sections and practices based on moderation in this book. They were written for you.

Reason five: we trust everyone but ourselves.

Are you constantly asking other people to write you a meal plan? Are you always trying to get free advice from somebody about your macronutrients? Are you constantly worried that you're not following the right diet based on somebody else's recommendations?

You're not trusting yourself. We are going to go over this one in depth in the nutrition chapter, so if this is you, stay tuned.

Lastly, reason six: we need a distraction.

So many times we are simply bored and looking for something to fixate on. Food and weight are easy fixations because they provide instant gratification.

We will cover this in detail in "The Part Where We Talk about Fasting."

But now let's talk about one of my favorite topics.

DISORDERED EATING AND SOCIAL MEDIA

Let's escape in a scenario for a moment, shall we?

It's a Friday night, and you have no plans. You decide it would be a great opportunity for you to snuggle up with your Netflix queue and enjoy a homemade healthy dinner.

Yes, tonight is the night you will be good.

You will be good and eat good, healthy food and finally start that diet you keep telling yourself needs to happen.

Putting on comfortable clothes, you turn on your television and start that movie you've watched a million times but just never get tired of, with a bowl of steamed broccoli and grilled chicken resting in your lap. After three minutes, the meal you spent 30 minutes preparing disappears.

Dang.

That wasn't very satiating.

Your antsy hands get restless so you start sifting through Instagram, looking at other people's dinners.

Amy is having a sushi date with her boyfriend of two years. It's their one cheat meal for the week.

Kayla is enjoying a "protein power bowl" with all the delicious toppings. Apparently, it fits her macros.

Denise is having a weird but delicious looking sugar-free, fat-free waffle and egg sandwich after her intense leg session. This is something she calls clean eating.

All of these beautifully fit people in their beautiful relationships eating their beautiful food.

You start thinking, *Well, maybe I should spend tonight finding out what my macros are. Then I can add more food into my dinner tonight because I'm still hungry and, this way, I can do it without feeling bad about it!*

So you pull up some phony macro calculator to figure out your daily caloric and macro needs. After pinpointing the number, you find a calorie and macro-counting app on your iPhone and start logging in all of the food you had that day.

Thirty minutes later, you've logged all of your food, though you feel a little guilty because you didn't weigh everything earlier in the day so you're not sure if you're entering the correct grams.

This thought eats away at you, but you try to ignore it and say you'll start fresh tomorrow.

That's right, you'll start fresh tomorrow. So, in actuality, you really deserve to eat whatever you want tonight.

Yes, yes, forget the calories and macro counting tonight; tomorrow the real diet starts, and so tonight you can really eat whatever.

You reach for the fat-free sweet potato chips you have on your top shelf, hidden far in the back. Cracking open the bag, you pour out all of the contents into a big bowl and begin to nosh.

Thirty minutes later, you feel terrible. You have guilt. You're angry. You're bloated and frustrated. You don't feel like you did what Kayla from Instagram must have done in order to get those crazy amazing abs she has.

You decide that you need to create an actual meal plan to follow tomorrow to ensure you stay on track.

An hour later, you have your diet planned perfectly, down to the last macronutrient gram.

Yes! You look at your clock and see it's midnight. Your night is gone.

But not before one more fat-free cookie…

And so the cycle continues.

How familiar does this situation sound?

Honestly, think about it. Have you been here before?

I know I sure have. And it's not easy. But here is what I have been able to gather from reflecting on these patterns.

We all have triggers. One of my triggers is comparison. Unfortunately, we live in a day and age where social media makes it extremely easy to compare in an instant.

Listen to me now.

Nobody's life is perfect. There is no reason you should waste a single moment of your beautiful life comparing your life to somebody else's life, and the same goes for diet. If Instagram and Facebook are contributing to how you structure your diet and eat your foods, then it's really time for you to make a huge decision.

I challenge you to make a choice. Decide for yourself to:

1. Delete your Instagram, Facebook, Pinterest, or what have you for one month.
2. Unfollow every account that triggers you.

This may sound extreme, but it's actually not. In fact, this is one of the best things I ever did for myself.

On top of unfollowing accounts, I actually stopped contributing to the fad. I very rarely take pictures of my food. I rarely check in anywhere about where I'm eating or who I'm with.

Now, I live in the moment.

I don't need "fans" to like my food. *I* need to like my food. Period.

I am the only person who matters when it comes to what I put in my body, and I hope more of us can start to see it that way.

Additionally, I no longer have nights where I make steamed broccoli and dry chicken breast. Why? Cause that's not what nourishes me. That's not what makes me satiated. It might for some people, but many people eat that simply because they're trying to restrict themselves for the sake of following some bogus diet.

Stop the comparison and naturally, you may learn to stop the dieting. Stop the dieting, and you'll stop the disordered eating.

This week, I implore you to accept my challenge.

Break the comparison-triggering link that's binding you to disordered eating.

Do it.

20 PRACTICES FOR BREAKING FREE

This. Right. Here.

Write these down. Print these off. Tattoo them to your thighs. I don't care where these 20 practices exist, all I care is that you know them and you remember them.

These 20 practices will help you break up with your disordered eating as you cultivate food freedom and unconditional body respect. Some of these we have already learned about, and some of these we will soon learn about, but if I know anything, it's that reiteration is a key player in transformation.

1) Don't diet.

That means no meal plans, calorie counting, macros, or off-limit foods. If you're allergic to something, that's different, but don't cut something out of your diet from fear or the desire to restrict.

2) Explore love.

The desire to binge eat or avoid eating altogether often leads to poor relationships with others and restricts social gatherings where you can meet others. Try dating or opening yourself up to new relationships. If you're already in a relationship, spice things up. Get creative.

3) Find a new hobby that's not related to food or physical exercises.

Learn a new language, pick up an instrument, make something with your hands, or grow a garden. Just find something to do that doesn't revolve around food or fitness.

4) Eat whatever you want whenever you want without limitations.

Yeah, that's scary. But do it. You'll discover that you are no less loved than before, and soon the forbidden foods will lose their magic.

5) Think about why you love those whom you love.

Is it because they're thin? Is it because of their abs or defined, long legs? No? I didn't think so. You love people for who they are on the inside, and people love you for the exact same reason.

6) Get a dog.

Seriously, I can't even explain how much dogs help you move past your body obsessions. All of a sudden, you have somebody to look after who might just become more important than your mission to create the perfect body. They make you smile, laugh, and love. They also make excellent cuddle buddies. Lastly, a dog will never love you any less for how to look.

7) Get the **** off social media.

Stop following accounts and pages that make you think you're any less perfect than you are. If you're addicted to looking at people who live lifestyles you wish you had, you're not doing yourself any favors. Unplug and start living.

8) Buy clothes that make you feel good.

Do you buy clothing that's too small for your current body, hoping it will encourage you to lose weight? Stop that. That does not encourage you to fulfill your amazing human potential, and it degrades your self-worth. You're *way more* than a size small or a size 4. Buy clothes that look good on you now because you *deserve* it.

9) Escape.

Sometimes we need to get away to de-stress and reprioritize, even if it's just to a bed and breakfast in the next town over. Stress can makes us want to control different aspects in life such as food, weight, or exercise. Escaping and relaxing can help all of us to calm down and give ourselves the care and attention we deserve. Go for a trip, small or large, and pamper your precious soul.

10) Trade the gym for outdoors for one month (at least).

If you've been working out in a gym for years and years, it's time for a break. If you work out solely for aesthetics-related reasons, it's time for a break. If you have a hard time putting anything else before the gym, it's time for a break. How we feel about our bodies is strongly related to our eating habits, stress levels, and overall health. Taking a break from the equipment and spending more time outdoors is greatly beneficial and, dare I say, *necessary*.

11) Incorporate yoga and meditation into your daily routine.

Yoga makes you slow down and appreciate your body's ability to move and balance. Meditation forces you to spare a few moments to stop what you're doing and reflect, relax, and simply *be quiet*. If you're the type of person who doesn't like slowing down and doing yoga, then you're most likely the exact type of person who would benefit from it the most. Just give it a try.

12) Compliment others more.

Seeing the beauty in others, making strangers smile, and being kind to your neighbor is extremely beneficial for your heart. Not only does it brighten their day, but it also improves yours.

13) Journal.

Journaling is a great way to express your thoughts, emotions, and feelings without having to put too much thought or effort into the writing process. It's actually best to not think about it at all but rather to write exactly what you want to at *that* very moment. You can also try blogging or video blogging if you want to share your experiences with others.

14) Say yes more.

It's really easy to get into the habit of saying no to things that sound like they will require too much effort, are too much out of our comfort zone, or will make you feel vulnerable. There are a million and one reasons not to do something, but it's up to you to recognize the one reason *to* do something. Go to the party, ride the horse, do the handstand, buy the book, and eat the food. Just try it. You may find yourself with a new passion, friend, or memory.

15) Enjoy more books, audiobooks, or podcasts in your spare time.

Instead of listening to music in the car, enjoy a podcast that will leave you feeling inspired and encouraged. Instead of watching TV at night, get lost in fiction. Try to avoid reading about the topic or subject that might be consuming your mind already (nutrition, fitness, health, etc.), but do read something that's totally frivolous and enjoyable. When you listen to podcasts, seek out ones that will give you valuable and useful information you can incorporate into your own life.

Here's a list of my favorite books (my first recommendation is *You Are a Badass*):

(http://www.mindbodymusings.com/books) And then check out my very own podcast **here**:

http://www.mindbodymusings.com/category/the-podcast

16) Throw away the scale.

Throw away the food scale and your body weight scale. You don't need either of them to live a happy, amazing life. In fact, they can often ruin the best of days for absolutely no reason at all. A food scale is good for understanding how to eyeball food at the *beginning*, but you have no reason for it after a few weeks. Your bathroom scale is pointless at all times. Improve your body based on your health and how you feel, not how much you weigh.

17) Sleep at least 8-10 hours a night.

You might need even more sleep than this. It's possible that you can function with less. But science shows without a doubt that sleep is directly correlated with quality of life and happiness. Start going to sleep just a little bit earlier, and make sure the quality is solid. If you're waking up several times throughout the night, take actions such as cultivating a more peaceful sleep environment, cutting back on the caffeine, or getting a sleep mask. Sleep is crucial for having an optimal mind-body relationship.

18) Say "thank you" when you receive compliments.

If somebody compliments you, don't you dare say, "This old thing?" or "Ugh, I've always hated my nose, but thanks." Instead, accept your compliment politely and show appreciation for their words. They meant their words, and whatever they said is true. So enjoy your compliment!

19) Wash your body with just your hands…and soap.

Skip the loofah. Washing your body with your own hands is a pretty intimate experience and can help you to appreciate your body on a daily basis. This is a habit I've developed over the past few years, and it's helped me to slow down and fully enjoy the simple pleasure of a hot shower.

20) Be more aware of self-talk.

If you're walking around all day telling yourself that you're not pretty, you're too big, you're stupid, you're a failure, then you're going to start believing it. *I repeat*: If you tell yourself something enough times, you *will* believe it. The same applies for positive self-talk. If you tell yourself over and over you're a success, you're amazing, you're worth more than what you weigh, you're in control, and you're perfectly made, then you *will* believe it. Start talking to yourself with kind words, encouragement, and love. This, above all, will improve your mind, body, and spirit connection.

Well, there you have it. And hopefully you *literally* have it, meaning these should be pinned up somewhere.

I mean it.

6

The Part Where We Talk About Fasting

One thing I do very often in my practice with clients is encourage them to create a Fasting and Feasting List.

No, this isn't the kind of fasting you're thinking of. I'm not talking about food; I'm talking about fasting from habits and rituals.

This list is actually something that helped me tremendously in my self-discovery journey. Here's what you do:

1. Pull out a pen and piece of paper.
2. Draw a line down the middle.
3. On the top of the left side write "Fast."
4. On the top of the right side write "Feast."

The next part is relatively easy to plan out, while managing to be surprisingly difficult to put into action.

On the side that says "Fast," I want you to write down all of the habits you know you should stop doing, and put some kind of timeframe on it. For example, mine said:

- Do not count macros for this entire year.
- Do not hire a diet or fitness coach to tell me how to eat for this entire year.
- Do not force myself to run sprints in the morning if I do not feel like it this year.

- Do not force myself to go to the gym six days a week this year.
- Do not force myself to eat chicken and broccoli anymore this year.
- Do not obsess over reading nutrition articles this year.

On the flip side, where it says "Feast," I want you to write down all of the habits you want to start creating. These do not necessarily need to have a time frame on them. For example, mine would say:

- Begin to take more walks outside.
- Start eating out with new friends once or twice a week.
- Experience mindful eating at least once every day.
- Read more fiction instead of non-fiction.
- Aim to go to sleep by 10:00 pm every night.
- Wake up by 6:00 am every morning (not to work out, but to work on business-related things).
- Habitually compliment other women about their inner beauty.

These were new habits that I knew were *realistic* for me to create; and notice that I don't have anything diet-related on this list.

My goal with these lists was to decrease the amount of time I spent thinking about food and fill it with more time doing things that will help me to grow as a person.

One thing that I have definitely learned in my coaching practice is that if you're going to try to take away a habit, you most certainly need to have something to replace it with. This list is a great visual of what new hobbies and activities you can implement in your day-to-day life. Don't choose things you'll never do, but choose serious passions that you have but keep pushing away.

Once your list is complete, hang it on your fridge, put it in your wallet, stick it to your mirror…just have it somewhere where you will see it each and every day.

Keep this paper out in the open for the next months to come and you will see how easy it is to remember to do the things you know you really love.

Not only will this help you create a better life for yourself, but it will also help you respect your own bio-individuality when it comes to nutrition.

7

Approaching Nutrition with Sanity in Mind

Talking about nutrition has become one of my least favorite things. It's not that I don't absolutely love nutrition and food; it's because I don't ever want to be a part of the noise.

You know, the noise where Billy Joe says paleo is the only way, even though Mary Lou says veganism is a life-changer, but yet Francis Ellen claims gluten-free is the only way to be.

I am never going to come to you and say "this" is the answer, and, vice versa, I will never say "this" *isn't* the answer.

My view on nutrition is pretty simple, and it can be summed up in one sentence: *It is not about doing what you think should work or what you hear works; it is about doing what actually works for YOU.*

Refuse to drink the Koolaid. Go against the grain. Be fearless with your choices. Be different. Be yourself.

In order to find out what actually works with your body, yes, there will be some trial and error involved. It is important to know how certain foods react in your body. It is extremely beneficial to have tried out different diets and know which ones made you break out, which ones made you miserable, which ones made you cranky, which ones were just too freaking difficult, and so on.

Let me repeat, that information IS useful and there is a time and a place for it, but once you have that knowledge, there is absolutely no reason to continue trying out the same diet over and over again if it makes you miserable.

The very first thing I do with my clients is challenge them to try intuitive eating. The book *Intuitive Eating* by Evelyn Tribole and Elyse Resch, is one of the most life-altering books I have ever read, and I recommend all of my clients read this book front to back.

In a nutshell, intuitive eating is eating what sounds good when you're hungry and stopping when you are full. For some people, being "hungry" and "full" might not be as obvious as it is to others, and that's okay.

We start there. I tell people to start eating what sounds good and eating until they are at a contentment level of about 8 on a 1-10 scale.

The second thing I have them do is journal their thoughts before and after their meals. What kind of things are they telling themselves before they eat?

"Work is so stressful, I need candy."

"My husband is so mean, I need to order a pizza."

"I love and respect myself so much, I need nourishment."

And then you journal the "after" thoughts.

"I can't believe I just ate a bucket of candy. I am going to be sick."

"I knew I shouldn't have ordered a large. Now I won't be able to think clearly until I finish the whole thing."

"I am so fortunate to have had the opportunity to eat that meal. I feel great and now I am going to move on with my life!"

These thoughts are tremendously eye-opening for many. Sometimes you don't know how foods make you feel until you write them down and actually see them on paper.

This is one side of the coin in regard to your relationship with your meals. The other side is how the food actually makes you *feel*, not what it makes you *think*.

As well as writing down their thoughts, I have my clients journal their experience.

- Do they have energy after eating?
- Do they have a stomachache?

- Do they have "audible" digestion?
- Is their skin breaking out?
- Are they ready for a nap?

These types of queries are really helpful when determining what foods work best with your body. People generally assume that you'll only know what foods work well with your body IF you try a diet, but the truth is, you can examine how you feel with certain foods after meals with them! It doesn't always have to be an all-or-nothing approach.

After examining your instant emotions as well as your bodily responses, then you can take the next steps. If meat is starting to slow down your digestion, maybe limit the meat a bit.

You don't have to become a vegetarian.

I repeat. You don't have to become a vegetarian.

Simply reduce the consumption.

Same goes for everything else. Does gluten give you anxiety? Then choose foods that don't contain gluten most of the time. You don't have to label yourself as gluten-free, but you can simply look for other options.

Does eating fat in the morning give you more energy? Great! You can eat fat in the morning as much as you feel like it…but again, you don't have to do that every single day.

Finding what works well for you means exactly that. You know what works *well* for you. What it DOESN'T mean is that you can never change up that plan and do something else. It means that you are now equipped with some great knowledge and can use it to your advantage as often or as little as you would like.

Do not get consumed with being "something-free." Whether it's meat-free, dairy-free, gluten-free, soy-free, seed-free, blue-things-free, red-things-free, and so on. In this all-or-nothing type culture, we're told to go balls to the wall on everything, and if we don't, we aren't accepted in that club.

Listen to me now. Your diet is not something you sacrifice for the sake of belonging to a diet club.

Truth be told, diet clubs are for shmucks, and you're way too good for that.

With that said, if you currently feel chained to a diet club and you're scared about losing that identity, then this part was written specifically for you. Your club friends are not really friends if they are actually going to be mad at you for doing what's right for your body instead of following food rules. On the flip side, if they continue to be your friend, well then, yay! You have good friends and a good diet now.

Moral of the story: Stop labeling yourself as "something-free" when you don't have to. **Just. Be. Free.**

Allergies are one thing. Sensitivities are one thing. Wanting to belong—that's a completely different thing.

Besides, after you finally stop labeling yourself and give yourself the freedom to intuitively eat food that makes you thrive, you'll be able to accomplish so much more in life. You'll be free from food distractions, and you'll have so many doors open!

Don't believe me?

Try it for yourself. You will see.

NUTRITION BASICS

Now that I've made it perfectly clear that moderation and balance is not only fine, it's GREAT, I want to give you some tips and guidelines that I personally use when I make my meals.

Some of these things might not resonate with you and if that's true, please skip them. They are not for everybody, but they will probably resonate with those of you who are a fan of balance. Hopefully that's you.

The 15 Principles of Balance:

1. Eat a lot of plants.
2. Don't limit anything from your diet.
3. Don't see food as "good" or "bad."
4. Don't plan indulgences OR restrictions.
5. Only count calories once in a blue moon (if you want) to make sure you're on the right track and not eating too little for your activity levels.
6. Eat when you're hungry and stop when you're full (mostly).
7. Never worry about what your next meal is going to be.
8. Never punish yourself after you eat something that's not green.
9. Don't typically eat foods that make you gassy or bloated (not during the day, at least).
10. Buy local when possible but don't give it a second thought if you can't make it work.
11. Sometimes eat foods that come from a package, but don't make that the bulk of your diet.
12. Eat breakfast if you're hungry, or wait if you're not.
13. Don't immediately act on advice from strangers about nutrition. Investigate for yourself and know what works from trial and error.
14. Don't read nutrition forums because that crap is contradictory.

15. Don't compare your food to anybody else's.

These are *principles* because these fifteen things come together to make your *own* diet work for you. You shouldn't have to "work hard" to do any of the things above, as they should come naturally and with ease.

Personally, these principles bring me joy, and they have helped me (and my clients!) discover what food truly makes our bodies feel great.

Let's take a deeper look, shall we?

1) *Eat a lot of plants.*

To make that a little clearer, let me say that I eat a lot of plants that I LIKE. It's true that I didn't always like green things, so initially I did do a bit of experimenting until I found the ones that I could tolerate, and I found the exact way I wanted to tolerate them. If you honestly don't like *any* vegetables right now, look up new recipes that involve cooking with different spices, oils, and seasonings. For example, you may kind of like broccoli, but not that much. Try sautéing broccoli in lots of butter. Then later on, decrease the butter a little and add some salt. Keep changing it around to see what you like best, and eventually, I bet you'll find something that you simply love.

2) *Don't limit anything from your diet.*

Back in the day, I was addicted to cutting out major food groups from my diet. No more carbs. No more meat. No more this or that. Now, I never limit ANYTHING. I am "allowed" to eat anything I want. (And no, there's no fine print to that!) If I begin to limit myself from something, it's naturally going to become the one thing that I want and, eventually, the one thing that I can't eat enough of. You may have experienced cutting something out of your diet and then finding yourself binging on it at one point. This is psychological. You don't know when you'll be able to have that food again so you want to eat all of it when you give yourself permission to have one little taste. I no longer have any binges because I no longer have any restrictions.

3) *Don't see food as good or bad.*

If I start to see food as good or bad, I will start to feel good or bad after eating said food. If I eat broccoli and chicken, I will allow myself to feel good. If I eat cake, I will allow myself to feel bad. If I feel bad, I will want to punish myself. The results of feeling bad can be extensive, including feelings of guilt, frustration, and anxiety. These emotions will lead me to want to "work off" the food on the treadmill, or maybe create a new meal plan for myself to follow so I don't ever get off track again. And the cycle continues. I no longer see food as good or bad, and, as a result, I never feel good or bad for my choices. Well, I actually do feel good but it's not BECAUSE of my food choices.

4) *Don't plan indulgences or restrictions.*

I never plan to have a "cheat meal." Similarly, I never plan to have a "diet" day. I eat the foods I like, and I eat them until I'm content. Life has unexpected events all the time; each day can be different. Some days I feel like a cheeseburger, and some days I feel like a lettuce wrap. Sometimes I eat light in the morning and feast at night. Sometimes I eat a huge breakfast in the morning and then just graze for the rest of the day. My activity levels change each day, my cravings change each day, the weather is different every day, and my schedule is always different. I don't plan to eat any particular way at any point, because if I do, I will experience guilt when I get off that "plan." Just forget the plans.

5) *Only count calories once in a blue moon to make sure you're on the right track and not eating too little for your activity levels.*

I'm not against counting calories. I'm really not. For some people, this works just fine, and they never let themselves get obsessed with it. For others, this is a coping mechanism for life. It's a way they manage stress. For me, I simply want to make sure I'm not burning more calories than I'm eating because I want to make sure that I have plenty of energy throughout the day. I no longer want to change my body because I love and respect it.

What I do want, however, is to make sure every day it's given what it needs. Once in a while, I will count my calories to make sure I'm in a good range, but one day is enough, and then I'm done.

6) *Eat when you're hungry and stop when you're full (mostly).*

I don't always eat when I'm hungry, and I don't always stop when I'm full. But for the most part, I can tell when I'm getting to the point where if I eat much more, I won't feel good. On the flip side, I know that around noon each day, I need to eat something because, if I don't, I will be too hungry by one o'clock and will want to overeat. I stay on top of my hunger levels so that I never get too hungry or too full, but I am not obsessed with it. For example, I eat whatever and whenever on holidays, and I will never change that.

7) *Never worry about what your next meal is going to be.*

If I'm busy worrying about what my next meal is going to be, then I'm going to be missing out on creating something amazing. I am going to be wasting precious hours of my life focusing on something that will come and will not fail me. I'm fortunate enough to have food whenever I need or want it so there's absolutely no reason to focus on controlling something hours in advance when I can just think about it later. Instead, I fill my time up with vastly more important things.

8) *Never punish yourself after you eat something that's not green.*

I do not discriminate. I'll eat white foods, brown foods, yellow foods, black foods, fat foods, skinny foods, short foods, tall foods. They all serve a purpose.

9) *Don't typically eat foods that make you gassy or bloated (not during the day at least).*

Like I said, I don't limit anything from my diet, but I'm smart about timing. For example, oatmeal sometimes makes me gassy, so therefore I don't eat it first thing in the morning when I have a CrossFit class and a full day of work ahead of me. I don't want to be uncomfortable in my office or at the squat rack. Instead, I save my yummy bowl of oats for later when I'm alone and don't have to worry about disrupting my friends. This is a win-win situation.

10) *Buy local when possible but don't give it a second thought if you can't make it work.*

Is local optimal? Sure, it's a great choice. At the same time, it's not the only choice. If I find local apples, then yes, I'll budget them in. But if it's between a regular non-local apple and a bag of "healthy" chips, I'm most likely going to choose the apple. It's not that I'm against the chips; it's just that I know apples bring me long-lasting nourishment whereas the chips might just deliver short-term satisfaction. Local or not, produce is produce is produce. Eat it.

11) *Sometimes eat foods that come from a package, but don't make that the bulk of your diet.*

My fridge is filled with fruits, vegetables, meats, and cheeses. My pantry contains packaged oatmeal, rice, beans, some protein bars, and some "healthified" cereals. *Gasp* *Madelyn, you eat cereal?!* Yes, as a matter of fact, I do. Sometimes I eat wheat. Sometimes I eat dairy. Sometimes I eat greens. I make sure that the bulk of my diet is considered "real food" (food that was grown, raised, or harvested) and then the other 10% is stuff that comes from a package that wouldn't necessarily be considered "whole foods." These percentages do not rule me, and I do not *follow* them. This is just what I typically do because I like it. I enjoy eating real foods, but I also enjoy sprinkling in some other things. To me, that's balance.

12) *Eat breakfast if you're hungry, or wait if you're not.*

I don't believe breakfast is mandatory for a good metabolism. I also don't believe that fasting in the morning is optimal. The only thing I believe is that my tummy is going to tell me what to do. Every morning is different. Therefore, I never plan in advance whether or not I'm going to eat breakfast. I simply wait and see.

13) *Don't immediately act on advice from strangers about nutrition. Investigate for yourself and know what works from trial and error.*

I am always open to listening and learning, but just because somebody claims carbohydrates cause brain fog doesn't mean it's true for me. If I'm interested enough, then I might test it out for a week or two. If I'm not interested, I will simply store that new information in my brain bank and save it for a rainy day.

14) *Don't read nutrition forums because that crap is contradictory.*

Just don't do this. If you're REALLY trying to find out information on something, read a study, book, or peer-reviewed journal. People that are on forums come from all different walks of life and have varying degrees of expertise. Billy Joe might have started paleo yesterday, yet he's already telling everybody that low carb is best and white rice is the devil. It would be really unfortunate if Francis Ellen read that and immediately took his word for it without doing research and ended up with metabolic damage and adrenal fatigue four months later. Just stay off nutrition forums.

15) *Don't compare your food to anybody else's.*

This is arguably the most important principle of all of my fifteen principles. I do not compare my diet to anybody else's. What I eat is my own business. I also try to keep my diet to myself instead of broadcasting it online, to keep anybody else from comparing their diet to mine. We all have different bodies and, therefore, different needs and tastes. Stop comparing your life, food, and body to others because you have no idea what's really going on in their lives, on the inside or the outside.

8

Stop Making Fitness So Complicated

Similar to nutrition, fitness can be taken to extremes. It can become an obsession, a comfort, and a distraction from life. On the flip side, it can be a life enhancer and a gateway to healthier decisions.

Fitness is not bad; in fact, it is a wonderful thing that can be used to your advantage, as long as you understand what fitness actually means.

Fitness means being healthy, so naturally you already know that rules out starvation and dieting.

YAY!

The trick behind fitness is choosing an activity and a way of movement that is pleasing and soothing to both your body and your soul.

For some people, that is CrossFit. For others, it is yoga. How do you know which one is for you? Simply put, you experiment. That's one of the beautiful parts about being free.

One of the number one reasons people quit their activity of choice is because they do not see immediate physical results. My challenge to you is to go into this seeking inner results, not outer results.

Experiment with a new fitness routine to see how it makes you *feel*, not how it makes you look. You may or may not see physical changes, and that's totally fine!

If you are really hoping to lose some weight, you will…but only once you find something that makes you happy. It doesn't have to be running or high-intensity cardio. People lose weight with yoga all the time. Do not force yourself to do any kind of activity that leaves you angry, frustrated, too tired to do anything else, or sad. Don't put yourself in an environment that makes you judge yourself. Don't force yourself to do anything that you hate. This should be common sense, but it's not. We think that "working out" is supposed to be boring and displeasing but au contraire! Working out might not be the most fun thing in the world, but moving your body, on the other hand, definitely is!

The best part about moving your body is that you can move your body in different ways every day! You don't have to dedicate your life to yoga and yoga alone. You don't have to only lift weights. You can do a combination of everything you love and create the movement schedule of your dreams.

For example:

- Monday: CrossFit
- Tuesday: Yoga
- Wednesday: Swimming
- Thursday: Take a walk!
- Friday: Resistance training
- Saturday: rest
- Sunday: rest

Instead of what you think you should do:

- Monday: CrossFit
- Tuesday: CrossFit
- Wednesday: CrossFit
- Thursday: CrossFit
- Friday: CrossFit
- Saturday: CrossFit
- Sunday: CrossFit

That will lead you down a dark path that will most likely end in a pulled shoulder and a slow metabolism.

Besides, picking only ONE type of movement and only sticking to that ONE type of movement is *so last year*. The way of the future is balance. The way of the future is diversity. Allow yourself to play around with all different types of sports and hobbies and activities!

My single and only rule for you is this: don't waste your time doing anything you hate! Life is way too short for that.

If you've been lifting weights in the gym for a couple years now and deep down you're sick of it, but you are just scared to stop doing it for reasons such as fear, worry, or anxiety, I CHALLENGE you to stop doing it and replace it with something new. You can even try taking walks instead! Allow yourself to change your program and do something that truly makes you happy.

I actually took an entire month off from any kind of physical activity besides walking in early 2014. I decided that I needed to divorce from my bodybuilding split routines because I felt chained to them. I felt like my identity was found within them, and I knew the only way I could break free was to literally break away.

That month was one of the biggest eye-opening experiences I ever had. My eating patterns improved, my mental health excelled, my mind-body love skyrocketed, my anxiety decreased, and I was finally able to discover that I was no longer in love with bodybuilding and that nothing happened once I stopped doing it.

I didn't get fat. I didn't lose my friendships. I simply gained happiness and more time in the day to do other things.

It was brilliant!

And after that month was over, I started searching for other activities that really did make me happy. I found a very happy medium at my local CrossFit gym where I can still enjoy my passion for lifting weights, but I am able to do it in a supportive group environment. I don't overwork myself by going every day, and I never, ever force myself to go if I don't feel up to it.

This month, you might need to take a break from something. Start searching for the types of activities that really make you thrive as a person. You should always leave your workout feeling refreshed and replenished, not drained and anxiety-ridden!

9

Becoming the Fearless, Confident, and Sexy Woman You're Meant to Be

As you begin your self-discovery journey and venture out into the world of practical health, you're going to be surrounded by people who are not "there yet," and that's okay. You might be the best example of true health that they will ever see. How powerful is that?

People are going to continue to complain about their body, life, relationships, food, and fitness, but that doesn't mean you have to join in.

Stand for what you believe in each and every day and routinely implement all of the different practices I have provided for you in this book. All of the lessons you have learned in this book will ultimately come together to give you the tools you need to experience your full potential.

- You ARE fearless.
- You ARE confident.
- You ARE sexy.
- You ARE beautiful.
- You ARE free.

You are everything you want to be. You have the capability to throw all of your food fears, body image struggles, and inner worries to the side and actively pursue the life of your dreams. You no longer need to let disordered eating rule your day-to-day schedule because you understand where your desire to control food comes from and you know how to work through it.

You know that freedom is possible and within your reach.

I hope you have enjoyed your time spent reading *The Perfection Myth,* and I certainly hope to connect with you in the future.

Warmly,

Madelyn Moon

Share the Love

Thank you so much for investing your time into this book. If you found *The Perfection Myth* to be insightful and full of knowledge, please take a moment to write a review on Amazon. Each review helps my book extend its reach and lets me tell others about unconditional body respect. I believe all of us could use more of that in our lives! Thank you so much!

The Next Step

Ready to take the next step? Hungry for more body love and food freedom?

I've created a free self-love "how-to" guide, which you can grab from my website.

Download **10 Proven Steps for Ending Any Diet Obsession** here: http://bit.ly/1F6DCqd

About the Author

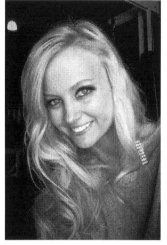

Madelyn Moon spent the last several years training for fitness competitions and modeling photo shoots, only to come to the conclusion that obsessing over food and her body was taking her further away from her passion, not closer. Today, Life Coach Maddy Moon teaches other women and men how to take control of their relationship with food while enjoying every minute of their newfound freedom.

Madelyn is the host of the Mind Body Musings Podcast and the creator of the site, maddymoon.com. She is a graduate from the University of Texas in Austin and the Institute for Integrative Nutrition and currently resides in Colorado, coaching clients online.

18076604R00038

Printed in Poland
by Amazon Fulfillment
Poland Sp. z o.o., Wrocław